BATTLING MIGRAINE

A Beginners Guide To Migraine: Diagnosis, Treatment, Coping & Living Well

ROGER ANDREW

Contents

Introduction

A migraine is a type of headache disorder characterized by recurrent, severe headaches that typically produce intense throbbing or pulsing pain on one side of the head. Migraines can also affect both sides of the head and occasionally induce facial or neck pain.

Migraines are frequently accompanied by additional symptoms, which can differ from person to person but can include the following.

• Sickness and vomiting.

• Light sensitivity (photophobia).

• Sound sensitivity (phonophobia).

• Some individuals experience visual disturbances, such as blinking lights or zigzag lines, prior to the onset of a headache. This is known as a migraine aura and is experienced by a subset of migraine sufferers.

Migraine attacks can range in duration from hours to days and can be incapacitating, making it difficult for individuals to carry out daily tasks. Migraines are believed to be caused by a combination of genetic, environmental, and neurological factors, but their precise origin is not completely understood.

There are numerous migraine varieties, including:

• Migraine without aura is the most prevalent form of migraine, characterized by a headache without preceding visual disturbances.

• Before experiencing a migraine with aura, some individuals experience specific visual, sensory, or motor disturbances. Auras are the name given to these disturbances, which typically last less than an hour.

• Chronic migraine is defined as migraines occurring 15 or more days per month for at least three months.

Migraines can be treated with a variety of methods, including lifestyle adjustments, avoidance of triggers, and medication.

During an attack, over-the-counter pain relievers like ibuprofen or prescription medications like triptans may be used to alleviate symptoms. Migraine sufferers who experience frequent or severe headaches may also be prescribed preventive medications.

It is essential for individuals with migraines to develop a personalized treatment plan that addresses their specific requirements and triggers in collaboration with healthcare professionals.

CHAPTER ONE
Factors And Reasons

Migraines can be triggered by a number of different factors, but their precise cause is still unknown. However, it is believed that genetic, neurological, and environmental factors are involved. Here are some of the most prevalent migraine triggers and possible causes:

• Migraines frequently run in families, indicating a genetic component to the disorder. If migraines run in your family, you may be more susceptible to developing them.

• Migraines can be triggered by hormonal fluctuations, particularly in women. Numerous women report experiencing migraines during their menstrual cycles, pregnancies, and menopause. Additionally, hormonal contraceptives can influence migraine frequency.

• High levels of tension and anxiety can cause migraines in some individuals. In addition, the "let-down" phase following a period of tension can trigger migraines.

• Dietary Factors: Certain foods and beverages are known to induce migraines in some individuals. Alcohol (especially red wine), caffeine, chocolate, aged cheeses, and foods containing MSG (monosodium glutamate) are common dietary triggers.

• Bright lights, loud noises, strong odors, and weather changes can induce migraines in certain individuals. Some individuals are susceptible to migraine attacks when exposed to flickering or blinking lights.

• Some individuals can experience migraines as a result of both insufficient and excessive slumber. A consistent sleep schedule can reduce the likelihood of developing migraines.

• Sometimes, intense physical activity or overexertion can induce migraines. This is commonly known as "exercise-induced migraines."

• As a side effect, certain medications, including certain vasodilators and oral contraceptives, can cause migraines. If you are taking medication, it is essential to discuss potential migraine triggers with your healthcare provider.

• Some individuals can develop migraines as a result of insufficient water consumption or dehydration.

• Sensory Stimuli: In migraine-prone individuals, bright or flickering lights, harsh sounds, and strong odors can trigger migraines.

• Changes in Routine: Migraines can be triggered in some people by sudden changes in their daily routines, such as avoiding meals or eating at irregular times.

• Allergic reactions or allergen exposure can sometimes trigger migraines in susceptible individuals.

It is essential to note that migraine triggers can vary significantly from person to person, and what causes a migraine in one person may not cause one in another. Identifying and managing specific migraine triggers is essential for prevention. Keeping a headache diary to record your activities, diet, and potential migraine triggers can be helpful in identifying their causes.

While these triggers can cause migraine attacks, it is important to recognize that they do not directly cause the underlying neurological changes that lead to migraines. Changes in blood flow, neurotransmitters, and nerve pathways, as well as other complex interactions within the brain, are the precise cause of migraines.

Migraine's fundamental mechanisms continue to be studied and comprehended with greater depth.

Frequent Symptoms

Migraine symptoms can differ between individuals and between migraine attacks. However, prevalent migraine symptoms include the following:

• The hallmark symptom of a migraine is a severe, pulsing or pulsating headache. It typically affects one side of the cranium, but both sides can be affected. Typically, the headache is accompanied by excruciating pain.

• Some people experience auras prior to the commencement of a migraine headache. Auras are typically visual aberrations, but they can also manifest as sensory or motor symptoms. Visions of flashing lights, zigzag lines, or blind areas are examples of common visual auras.

• Many people with migraines experience nausea, which can range from moderate discomfort to severe sickness. During a migraine assault, vomiting is possible.

• Sensitivity to Light (Photophobia): Even normal indoor lighting can aggravate migraine symptoms.

Migraine sufferers frequently find alleviation in dark or dimly lit rooms.

• Sensitivity to Sound (Phonophobia): During a migraine attack, loud disturbances or even normal-level sounds can be intolerable.

• Sensitivity to Smells (Osmophobia): During a migraine attack, certain odors can induce or aggravate migraines.

• During a migraine attack, physical activity or routine movements may exacerbate the headache discomfort.

• Even after the headache subsides, migraines can leave individuals feeling extremely exhausted and exhausted.

• During a migraine attack, some individuals experience disorientation or a spinning sensation (vertigo).

• Difficulty Concentrating: Migraines can impair cognitive function, making it challenging to concentrate or think effectively.

• Neck Pain Stiffness or distress in the neck is a symptom experienced by some migraine sufferers.

• In addition to visual disturbances, auras can cause sensory symptoms such as tingling or paralysis in the face or limbs, as well as motor symptoms such as weakness or difficulty speaking.

It's crucial to note that not all migraine sufferers experience auras, and not every migraine attack includes all of these symptoms. Migraines can differ in length and intensity. Some individuals may experience brief, mild attacks, while others may experience lengthier, more incapacitating ones.

If you suspect you have migraines or are experiencing severe headaches accompanied by any of these symptoms, it is imperative that you consult a healthcare professional for a proper diagnosis and to devise a treatment plan that is tailored to your needs. Effective management typically involves identifying and averting triggers, modifying one's lifestyle, and taking prescribed medications.

CHAPTER TWO
Migraine Analysis

Typically, migraines are diagnosed through a comprehensive medical evaluation conducted by a primary care physician or neurologist. The diagnosis is based on the patient's medical history, a detailed description of their symptoms, a physical examination, and, in some cases, additional tests to rule out other potential headache causes. Here are the diagnostic procedures for migraines:

• The medical professional will inquire about your headache symptoms, including their frequency, duration, and characteristics. Be prepared to describe the onset of your headaches, any accompanying symptoms (such as vertigo, vomiting, or light sensitivity), and any potential triggers or patterns you've observed.

• Physical Examination: A physical examination will be conducted to look for neurological abnormalities and other symptoms that may indicate an underlying medical condition.

• Diagnostic Criteria: To aid in the diagnosis of migraines, physicians frequently refer to diagnostic criteria established by the International Headache Society (IHS) or the American Migraine Foundation. The criteria may include the frequency, duration, and specific attributes of the affective condition.

• Since various types of headaches and other medical conditions can mimic migraine symptoms, your healthcare provider will want to rule out other possible causes. If there are atypical features or concerning neurological findings, additional tests such as blood tests, imaging studies (such as MRI or CT scans), or a lumbar puncture (spinal tap) may be necessary.

• Keeping a headache diary can be useful for documenting your symptoms, potential triggers, and the frequency of your headaches. It can provide your doctor with more information about your headache patterns.

• Discussion of Aura: If you experience auras before your migraines, provide detailed information about these visual, sensory, or motor disturbances. This can aid in the classification and diagnosis of migraines with aura.

• Mention if you have a family history of migraines because the condition has a genetic component.

After gathering all necessary information and ruling out other potential causes, your healthcare provider can diagnose migraine. On the basis of the characteristics of your headaches, the specific form of migraine (migraine with aura or migraine without aura) will be identified.

It is crucial to have a precise and precise diagnosis, as it guides treatment decisions. Migraines may be treated with lifestyle adjustments, the identification and avoidance of triggers, acute medications (to assuage pain during an attack) and preventive medications (to reduce the frequency and severity of migraines).

If you suspect you have migraines or are experiencing severe headaches with associated symptoms, seek medical attention immediately. A healthcare provider can assist you in effectively managing your condition and enhancing your quality of life.

Triggers For Migraines And Lifestyle Alterations

Migraine triggers can vary from person to person, but many migraine sufferers have identified common migraine triggers. Identifying and managing your specific migraine triggers can reduce their frequency and severity. Here are a few frequent migraine triggers and lifestyle modifications that may be helpful:

• High levels of stress can induce migraines in many individuals. It is possible for stress management techniques to reduce the impact of tension on migraine attacks. Consider mindfulness meditation, deep breathing exercises, yoga, and progressive muscle relaxation.

• Patterns of Sleep: Irregular sleep patterns, including insufficient and excessive sleep, can induce migraines. Maintain a regular sleep schedule, strive for 7 to 9 hours per night, and create a comfortable sleeping environment.

• Certain foods and beverages can cause migraines in some people. Alcohol (especially red wine), caffeine, chocolate, aged cheeses, and foods containing MSG (monosodium glutamate) are common dietary triggers. To identify your personal triggers, keeping a food journal can be beneficial.

• Migraines can be caused by dehydration, which can result from insufficient water consumption. Consume copious amounts of water throughout the day and limit your alcohol and caffeine intake, as these substances can contribute to dehydration.

• Skipping Meals Skipping meals or leaving for extended periods of time without eating can cause migraines. Consume regular, well-balanced meals to maintain stable blood sugar levels.

• Migraines can be triggered by hormonal fluctuations, particularly in women. If you observe a pattern of migraines related to your menstrual cycle, consult your healthcare provider about hormonal management options.

• Sensory Stimuli: In migraine-prone individuals, bright or flickering lights, harsh sounds, and strong odors can trigger migraines. If possible, avoid or reduce exposure to these stimuli.

• Changes in the weather, such as variations in barometric pressure or extreme temperature fluctuations, can induce migraines in some individuals. Although you cannot control the weather, being aware of its potential effects can help you prepare and take precautions.

• Physical Activity: Physical exertion or intense physical activity can sometimes induce migraines. Consider low-impact activities or a consistent exercise routine with progressive warm-ups and cool-downs if exercise is a trigger for you.

• As a side effect, certain medications, including certain vasodilators and oral contraceptives, can cause migraines. If you are taking medication, discuss potential migraine triggers with your healthcare provider.

• Alcohol and Caffeine: Although moderate alcohol consumption may be tolerated by some migraine sufferers, excessive alcohol consumption or specific types of alcohol, such as red wine, can provoke migraine attacks. Caffeine withdrawal can also induce migraines in some individuals, so if you consume caffeine frequently, try to maintain a consistent intake and avoid abrupt changes.

Migraine management typically involves identifying and avoiding triggers, maintaining a healthy routine, employing stress management techniques, and modifying diet based on individual triggers.

Additionally, if migraines are significantly impacting your quality of life, your healthcare provider may recommend medications for acute relief or prevention, and they can provide guidance on their use.

Keep in mind that it may take time and experimentation to identify your specific migraine triggers and determine the most effective lifestyle adjustments for managing your migraines. Keeping a migraine diary to record your symptoms, activities, and potential triggers can be a useful tool. Additionally, consulting with a healthcare provider or migraine specialist can provide you with individualized advice and treatment options.

CHAPTER THREE
Pharmaceuticals And Therapeutics

There are a variety of medications and treatment methods available for migraine management, ranging from acute pain alleviation to preventative measures.

The treatment you receive will depend on the frequency, severity, and unique characteristics of your migraines, as well as your medical history and specific requirements. Here is an overview of prevalent migraine medications and treatments.

1.   Acute   (Abortive) Pharmaceuticals:

• Over-the-Counter (OTC) Pain Relievers: When consumed at the onset of a migraine attack, OTC pain relievers such as ibuprofen, naproxen sodium, and aspirin can provide pain relief.

• Triptans: These prescription drugs, including sumatriptan, rizatriptan, and zolmitriptan, are designed specifically to treat migraines. They function by constricting blood vessels and obstructing brain pain pathways.

• Ergotamines: Ergotamine nasal mists and injections, such as dihydroergotamine (DHE), are sometimes used to treat severe migraines.

2. Preventative (Prophylactic) Drugs:

• Prescription Medications: If you experience frequent, severe, or debilitating migraines, your healthcare provider may prescribe preventive medications.

These include, among others, beta-blockers (such as propranolol), anticonvulsants (such as topiramate), tricyclic antidepressants (such as amitriptyline), and anti-CGRP monoclonal antibodies (such as erenumab, fremanezumab). The purpose of these medications is to reduce the frequency and severity of migraine attacks.

• Botox (OnabotulinumtoxinA): Botox injections may be prescribed for chronic migraines (15 pain days or more per month). Botox is injected into specific muscles of the head and neck to prevent migraines.

• Calcitonin Gene-Related Peptide (CGRP) Inhibitors: These newer medications, such as erenumab, fremanezumab, and galcanezumab, target CGRP, a protein linked to migraine attacks. Injections are administered monthly or quarterly.

3. First-Aid Medication:

• If acute medications are ineffective or migraines become too severe, your healthcare provider may prescribe rescue medications, such as nonsteroidal anti-inflammatory drugs (NSAIDs), corticosteroids, or anti-nausea drugs.

4. Behavioral and lifestyle approaches:

• Identifying and Avoiding Triggers: As stated previously, identifying and avoiding personal migraine triggers can be an integral part of migraine management.

• Establishing a regular sleep schedule, maintaining a balanced diet, staying hydrated, and managing tension with relaxation techniques can help reduce migraine frequency.

• Biofeedback and Relaxation Therapy: These techniques can help people learn to control their physiological responses to stress and tension, thereby decreasing the frequency and severity of migraines.

• Cognitive-Behavioral Therapy (CBT): CBT can be advantageous in managing the psychological aspects of migraines, such as anxiety and depression.

5. Alternative Medications:

• Alternative treatments, such as acupuncture, chiropractic care, herbal supplements, and dietary modifications, provide migraine relief for some individuals. Before pursuing alternative treatments, it is essential to consult with a healthcare professional to ensure that they are safe and appropriate for your specific situation.

6. Transcranial magnetic stimulation (TMS) devices and external trigeminal nerve stimulation (eTNS) devices are examples of medical devices designed to treat migraines or provide relief during an attack. These should be used under the supervision of a medical professional.

It is essential to work closely with a healthcare provider, preferably one with experience in migraine management, to develop a personalized treatment plan that meets your specific requirements.

This plan may include a combination of medications, lifestyle changes, and other therapies to effectively manage your migraines and enhance your quality of life. Consider that migraine management may necessitate some trial and error in order to determine the most effective treatment strategy for your specific situation.

Adaptive Strategies

Managing migraines can be difficult, but there are a number of strategies and lifestyle modifications that can help you manage your condition and enhance your quality of life. Listed below are some strategies for managing migraine afflictions:

1. Recognize and Evade Triggers:

• Keeping a migraine diary can help you identify specific migraine triggers that contribute to your attacks. After identifying triggers, you should take measures to avoid or reduce your exposure to them.

2. Create a Regular Routine:

Even on weekends, adhere to a regular sleep schedule by going to bed and rising up at the same time every day.

Consume well-balanced meals at regular intervals to prevent fluctuations in blood sugar.

• Stay well-hydrated by consuming enough water throughout the day.

3. Stress Administration:

• Employ techniques for reducing tension, such as mindfulness meditation, deep breathing exercises, progressive muscle relaxation, and yoga.

• Consider incorporating relaxation techniques into your daily routine, even when you do not have a migraine, in order to build stress resistance.

4. Dietary Modifications:

• Determine the foods and beverages that provoke your migraines and avoid them. Alcohol, caffeine, chocolate, aged cheeses, and foods containing MSG are common dietary triggers.

• Choose a diet abundant in fruits, vegetables, whole cereals, and lean protein.

5. Some individuals may experience migraines if they are dehydrated. Ensure you consume sufficient water throughout the day to maintain hydration.

6. Routine Exercise:

• Regular moderate exercise can reduce the frequency and severity of migraine attacks. However, excessive or intense physical activity can induce migraines in some individuals and should be avoided.

7. Medication Administration:

• Develop a medication management plan together with your healthcare provider. This may include acute medications to alleviate pain during migraine attacks or preventative medications to reduce the frequency and severity of migraines.

8. Verbal exchange:

• Be candid with your healthcare provider about your migraine symptoms, the efficacy of your treatment, and any adverse effects or concerns you may have.

• Inform your family, friends, and colleagues about your condition so that they can offer support and compassion during migraine attacks.

9. Create an Environment Friendly to Migraines:

• During a migraine attack, create a calm, dark, and comfortable space where you can retreat. Use blackout curtains, earplugs, and an eye cover to minimize sensory stimuli.

• Communicate your need for a calm environment during migraines to those around you.

10. Over-the-Counter Soothing:

• Keep over-the-counter pain relievers (such as ibuprofen or naproxen) on board for use in the early stages of a migraine attack, as they can be more effective if taken early.

11. Assistance Groups:

• Consider joining a migraine support group or searching for online communities where you can connect with people who understand your situation and share coping techniques and advice.

12. Professional Assistance:

• If you find it difficult to manage your migraines on your own, you should consider consulting a therapist or counselor. CBT can be effective for managing the psychological aspects of migraines.

13. Restricted Medication Use:

• Excessive use of pain-relieving medications can result in medication-overuse migraines. Consult your physician regarding the appropriate use of medications.

Keep in mind that discovering effective coping mechanisms may require trial and error. It is crucial to collaborate closely with your healthcare provider to develop a personalized migraine management plan that addresses your unique requirements and triggers.

You can better manage your migraines and reduce their impact on your life by implementing these strategies and seeking appropriate support.

CHAPTER FOUR
The Psychological Effects Of
Migraines

Migraines can have a substantial emotional impact on those who suffer from them. Migraines can result in a variety of emotional and psychological challenges due to the pain, unpredictability, and disruption they cause in daily life. Here are some emotional aspects and consequences of migraines:

• Migraine-related excruciating pain can cause significant distress, anxiety, and dread. Migraine attacks can be incapacitating and leave sufferers feeling impotent and overpowered.

• Anxiety and Anticipation: Many individuals with migraines experience anxiety and anticipation about when the next migraine attack will occur. This persistent concern about when the pain will occur can contribute to chronic anxiety and stress.

• Migraines are frequently associated with an increased risk of depression. The chronic nature of migraines, as well as the pain and limitations they inflict, can result in feelings of sadness, hopelessness, and depression.

• Isolation: Migraine attacks can result in social isolation. During an attack, people must frequently retreat to a dark, quiet room, which can contribute to feelings of social withdrawal and isolation. In addition, the dread of having a migraine in public or during social events can limit participation in social activities.

• Migraines can strain relationships with family members, friends, and employees. The inability of loved ones to completely comprehend the impact of migraines can lead to frustration and strained relationships.

• Frequent migraines can result in missed days of work or school, decreased productivity, and financial strain. This may lead to feelings of remorse and inadequacy.

• Migraines can substantially diminish a person's overall quality of life. Once-enjoyed activities may become difficult or impossible to engage in, resulting in a diminished sense of fulfillment and life satisfaction.

• Migraine Stigma: There is still a degree of stigma associated with migraines, with some people dismissing them as "just a headache." This lack of comprehension can add to the emotional burden, as individuals may feel invalidated or misunderstood.

• Migraine sufferers frequently develop effective coping strategies, but they may also experience frustration and fatigue as a result of perpetually managing their condition.

• Some migraine medications, especially preventive medications, can have adverse effects that affect mood and emotions. It is imperative to discuss any mood alterations with a healthcare provider.

It is crucial to recognize and address the emotional impact of migraines, as unaddressed emotional distress can exacerbate the condition and have a negative impact on overall health. Here are some measures to assist in coping with the emotional aspects of migraines:

• Seek Support: Discuss the emotional challenges associated with migraines with a therapist, counselor, or support group for assistance.

• Educate Yourself and Others: Learn more about migraines and share information with family and friends to help them better comprehend the condition.

• Communicate with your healthcare provider about the physical and emotional components of your migraines.

• Engage in Stress Reduction: To reduce anxiety and tension, engage in relaxation techniques, mindfulness, and stress management strategies.

• Lifestyle Management: Implement changes to your lifestyle to reduce migraine triggers and enhance your overall health.

• Medication Management: Work with your healthcare provider to identify the most appropriate medications and remedies to help you manage your migraines and the emotional distress they cause.

Remember that you are not alone in experiencing the emotional effects of migraines, and that seeking support and treatment can make a substantial difference in your ability to manage the condition.

Preventive Actions

Migraine preventive measures are strategies and treatments designed to lessen the frequency, severity, and duration of migraine attacks.

Even with the use of acute medications, these measures are notably beneficial for individuals who experience frequent or debilitating migraines. Changes in lifestyle, medications, and other interventions may be employed in preventive strategies.

The following are some common preventive measures for migraines:

1. Medical treatments:

• Prescription Migraine Prevention Medications: If you suffer from frequent, severe, or chronic migraines, your healthcare provider may prescribe migraine prevention medications. These consist of:

• Beta-blockers (propranolol, metoprolol, etc.).

• Anticonvulsants (for instance, topiramate and valproate).

• Tricyclic antidepressants (for instance amitriptyline).

• Calcium channel inhibitors (such as verapamil).

• Anti-CGRP monoclonal antibodies (e.g., erenumab, fremanezumab, galcanezumab).

• Botox (onabotulinumtoxinA) injections for chronic migraines.

Botox injections are an effective preventative treatment for chronic migraines. They are administered by a healthcare professional every 12 weeks.

2. Behavioral Modifications:

• Identify and Avoid Triggers: Keep a detailed migraine diary to identify and avoid your specific triggers, including specific foods, beverages, stressors, and environmental factors.

• Maintain a consistent sleep schedule by going to bed and rising up at the same time every day, including the weekends.

• Dietary Modifications: Avoid known dietary triggers and consume a well-balanced diet. Maintain adequate hydration and avoid postponing meals.

• Stress Management: Participate in stress-reduction techniques such as yoga, progressive muscle relaxation, and meditation.

• Moderate Exercise: Regular, moderate exercise can reduce the frequency and severity of migraines.

• Hydration: Maintain adequate hydration by consuming sufficient water throughout the day.

• Reduce or eliminate excessive caffeine and alcohol consumption, as these substances can induce migraines.

3. Avoid Excessive Medication Use:

• Use pain relievers with caution, as excessive use can result in medication-overuse migraines (rebound headaches). Follow your doctor's instructions regarding medication use.

4. Behavior Modification:

•	Cognitive-Behavioral Therapy (CBT): CBT can help individuals manage migraine-related stress, anxiety, and depression. It teaches coping techniques and relaxation methods.

•	Biofeedback and Relaxation Training: These therapies can help individuals learn to control their physiological responses to stress and tension, potentially reducing the frequency of migraine attacks.

5. Environmental Triggers to Avoid:

• Take measures to reduce your exposure to environmental triggers such as bright lights, loud sounds, strong odors, and weather variations.

6. Hormone Regulation (for Women):

• Women with migraines associated with their menstrual cycle may benefit from hormonal management strategies, such as birth control or hormone therapy. Consult a healthcare professional for available options.

7. Maintain Consistent Follow-Ups:

• Stay in close contact with your healthcare provider to monitor your migraine frequency and treatment effectiveness. Your preventive plan may require modifications over time.

It is essential to collaborate closely with a healthcare provider to develop a personalized migraine management plan that integrates the most effective preventive measures for your particular situation. The effectiveness of these measures can vary from individual to individual, and it may take time to discover the optimal combination of treatments and lifestyle modifications for you. Consistent communication with your healthcare team and a commitment to migraine management can result in significant enhancements to your quality of life.

Conclusion

Migraines are a complex and frequently incapacitating neurological condition characterized by severe headaches, frequently accompanied by additional symptoms such as nausea, vomiting, sensitivity to light and sound, and in some cases auras, which are visual disturbances. It is not completely understood what causes migraines, but genetic, neurological, and environmental factors are suspected.

Migraine management is a multifaceted process involving the identification of migraine triggers, lifestyle modifications, acute and preventive medications, and a variety of coping strategies.

Changes in lifestyle, such as adhering to a regular sleep schedule, managing stress, staying hydrated, and avoiding known migraine triggers, can significantly reduce the frequency and severity of migraine attacks. Both acute and preventative medications can provide respite during attacks and aid in preventing future episodes.

Significant emotional effects of migraines include anxiety, depression, social isolation, and relationship distress. It is imperative to address the emotional aspects of migraines and to seek support from healthcare professionals, therapists, and support groups.

Finding the most effective treatment for migraines is a highly individualized process that may require time and perseverance. Regular communication with a healthcare provider and a proactive approach to migraine management can significantly improve a person's quality of life and assist them in regaining control over their condition.

THE END

9 7 9 8 8 6 5 2 3 1 2 7 1